WEEDS

JOSEPH BAHRIBEK

WEEDS

iUniverse books may be ordered through booksellers or by contacting:

iUniverse
1663 Liberty Drive
Bloomington, IN 47403
www.iuniverse.com
844-349-9409

Because of the dynamic nature of the Internet, any web addresses or links contained in this book may have changed since publication and may no longer be valid. The views expressed in this work are solely those of the author and do not necessarily reflect the views of the publisher, and the publisher hereby disclaims any responsibility for them.

ISBN: 978-1-6632-2787-4 (sc)
ISBN: 978-1-6632-2788-1 (e)

Library of Congress Control Number: 2021916925

Print information available on the last page.

iUniverse rev. date: 01/19/2022

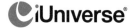

Introduction

I wrote this book for my love for weeds. I love weeds because they remind me of when used to walk in the <u>wilderness</u> in my home country. There were many weeds, some were nomadic on my way, and reminded me of St. John's, who used to walk along the wilderness and see many different weeds, this is why I chose to write a book about weeds, to commemorate St. John Baptist life. Wilderness and the variety of weeds he encountered.

J. E. B.

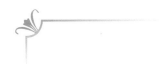

Alfalfa ???

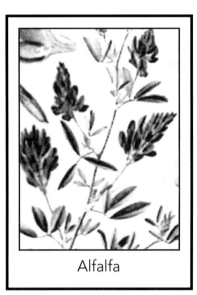

Alfalfa

Alfalfa (Medicago Sativa), also called Lucern, is a perennial flowering plant in the Legume family Fabaceae. It is cultivated as an important forage crop in many countries around the world. It is used for grazing, hay, and silage, as well as a green manure and cover crop. The name alfalfa is used in North America. The name Lucern is more commonly used name in the United Kingdom, South Africa, Australia and New Zealand. The plant superficially resembles Clover (a cousin in the Sam family). Especially while young when trifoliate leaves comprising round leaflets are elongated. It has cluster of small purple flowers followed by fruits spiralled in 2 to 3 turns containing 10-20 seed. Alfalfa is native to warmer temperate climates. It has been cultivated as livestock fodder since at least the era of the ancient Greeks and Romans. Alfalfa sprouts are common ingredient in dishes made in South Indian cuisine.

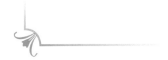

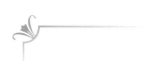

Aramanth

As the name suggests, chickweed makes a good green food for poultry, and also for pigs, it's useful as a feed to animals that have to be confined to a pen. A path of chickweed can be cut several times in a growing season. It can be added to salads or lightly steamed as vegetable.

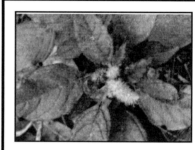

Aramanth

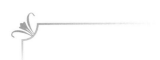

Green Aramanth

Now hailed as super green. Aramanth is a nutritious weed also known as pig weed. Common weeds on lighter soils such as in East Anglia and often appear where the soil is enriched, for example by big manure, which may be why it is also called pigweed. It is a very good food source for birds, who loves seeds, but we can eat it too. Aramanth is another edible green, quite mild in flavour and usually found in the warmer months. In Greece it is cooked and dressed with olive oil and lemon juice, and it's common food in South India. The seed are small, but they are said to be high in protein, and there are various recipes for making a porridge from them Aramanth; it's suggested that it might replace kale as trendy vegetable for chefs steam or blanch it don't, cook it for long and serve it like spinach.

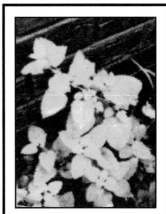

Green Aramanth

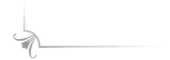

Asteroideae

Asteroideae is a subfamily of plant family Asteroideae, it contains about 70% of the Sepecies. The family is made of several tribes, including Astereae, Calenduleae, Eupetorieae, Cnaphalieae Heliantheae, Senecioneae and Tageteae. Asterideae contains plant found all over the world, many of which are shrubby. There are about 1.135 genera and 17,200 species within this subfamily; the large general by number of species are Helichrysum (500-600) and Artemisia (550) Asteroidiea

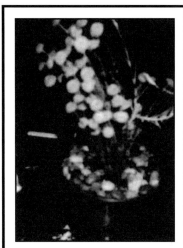

Asteroideae

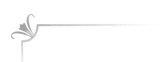

Bulbous Bluegrass

This common European weed is typical weed short leaves. It grows mostly frequently in dry area, and alone road side. This grass has the unusual ability to produce bublets rather than or in addition to seeds. This allows rapid production hostile environments where seedling would have difficulty becoming established juvenile plants beginning to develop from the bulbets stal on the plant. Ultimately they drop to the ground an establish themselves as independent plant. This common European weed. Short leaves. It grow most frequently in dry, gravel west and along roadsides.

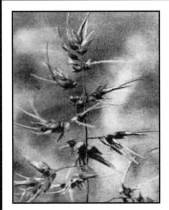

Bulbuos Bluegrass

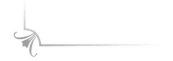

Green Bristlegrass

The tufted annual 1 to 2 feet tall the leaves are flat and rather short. Usually 2 to 3 per stem the common and Latin name describe the diagnostic fruiting Sike Setameans bristle Viridis mean green. The flowers and grains are densely clustered into 2 to 4 inch long green Spike covered with short bristles. This native of Eurasia is common weed in much of North American growing in waste areas and cultivated field. It is especially abundant along roadside.

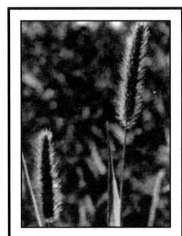

Green Bristlegrass

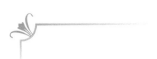

Creeping thistle

One or two other thistle can turn up in gardens occasionally but creeping thistle is the only one that is likely to be a serious problem common everywhere, this thistle spring up on posture, stream banks and roadsides at Woodlande, in waste space and garden and on all soils. The spreading the roots maybe found at least a few feet below the surface and the plant can regenerate from even small fragment. Creeping thistle can also spreads by seed.

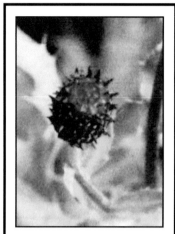

Creeping Thistle

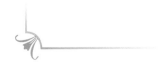

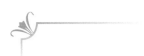

Lessertrefoil White Clover

The stem of these related and perfectly adapted lawn weed creep along below the mower blades. White clover spread by stolons, or runner, that root as they grow. In a fertile soil with no competition, one single shoot produced 157 feet (48m) of stolons in year, although they don't achives anything like that in the average lawn. Lessertrefoil also creep, but is an annual and grows from a single root. Both produce abundant, long-lived seed.

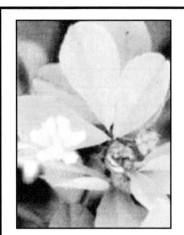

Lessertrefoil
White Clover

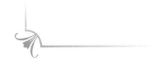

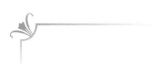

Cocklebur

Cocklebur xanthium is a coarse tall weed. Its chief claim to farm is it seed which are encased in burrs covered with hooked spines that often become entangled in with animal hair the burrs can reduce the value of sheep fleece, however cocklebur has a place in scientific history.

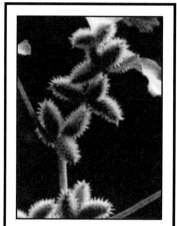

Cocklebur

Goosefoot

Goosefoot's cultivated cousin is C. Bouus henricus is a perennial called Good King Henry, a rather rare vegetable that sometimes appears on market stalls and the leaves can be picked continually through the summer. It looks similar to goosefoot.

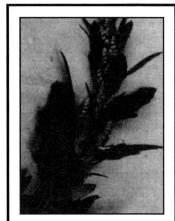

Goosefoot

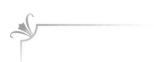

Common Mallow

The annual to sort lived perennial herb has long and taproot. The extensively branched stems spread over the ground. The leaves have long stalks and roundish to broadly heart shaped blades that are coarsely toothe and shallowly lobed. Common mallow introduced from Europe has spread to North America.

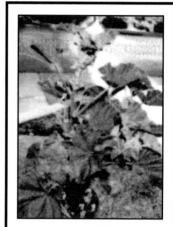

Common Mallow

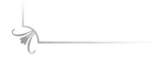

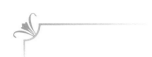

Cocklebur

Is a coarse and leafy grow to six feet. The alterate leaves have long stalks. Leaf blades are more or less heart-shaped, 2-6 inches long and wide and generally shallowily lobed with conspicuously toothed margins. Minutes bristly hairs do the stem and leaves the plant produce male and female flower. Male two seed female head have 2 disc flower. Cocklebur is native plant grow along roadside in West poison weed.

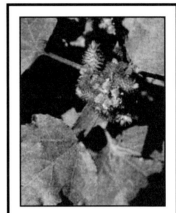

Cocklebur

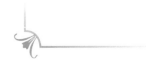

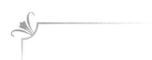

Cheat Grass

Is an annual weed, approximately one foot tall. Covered by soft (downy) hair. Each plant has two to several erect but arched stem bearing pendant spikelets which became most numerous in rich, moist soil. As growing conditions deteriorate the number of spikelets decreases. This ensures that plant resources are sufficient to produce at least a few fully developed seed. This European in Western North America in West.

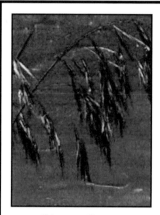

Cheat Grass

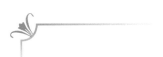

Crab Grass

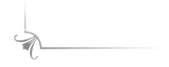
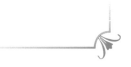

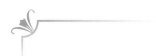

Curly Dock

Curly Dock is most widespread Rumex tall up to three feet tall. The weed is European the flower clusters, soft spiny margins. It is also introduced and abounds in moist areas, especially pastures. It is a robust perennial herb, up to three feet tall that crows from a stout taproot. The leaves are narrow (1 to 2 inches) and strap-like with grisp, curly edges. The upper leaves are smaller than those below. The stem are unbranched up many elongate flower clusters. The petal have a grain-like enlargement centered toward their base. This European weed is now widely established in cultivated field and pastures and occasionally invades rangelands broadleaf dock Rumex obtusifolius is a robust weed that closely resembles Curly Dock

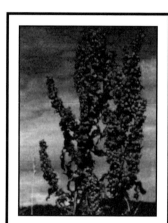

Curly Dock

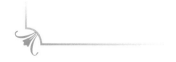

– C –

Cut ear

This weed is often mistaken for a dandelion even though the two species are clearly distinct. Both have only basal leaves but those of ear cut-ear are densely hairy, thus the common name. Also the tough and branched stems of cut-ear produs more than one head finall, the involucral bracts are narrow and the outer ones do not curve downward as in dandelions. The ear-cut grow in similar but more restricted habitats than dandelion. It is a terrible nuisance in lawns because of its weed appearance, and because the thick rosette of basal leaves smother the grass. It is especially abundant. West of the Cascada Rang, from Canada to California, perhaps the most conspicuous pasture and roadside weed during late summer. It is native of Europe.

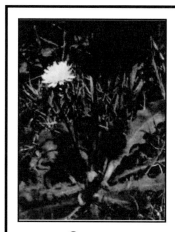
Cut ear

Chick Weed

The pioneer will pave the way for shallower root weed such as chickweed (Stellaria media), which will cover the ground so well that it won't dry out. Chick weed will also tend to smother other weeds, chickweed likes shady and moist conditions. A patch of chickweed can be cut several time in growing season.

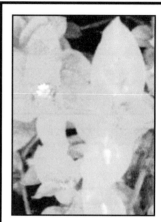

Chic Weed

White Clover

Wild White Clover (Trifolium repent) with its three, or rarely four round leaves, also contributes nitrogen. This is a small ground-hugging plant. It's a weed in lawns of course like many other useful plants the white or pinkish flower can be found between and October.

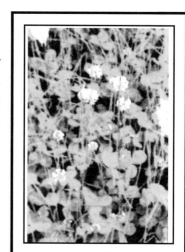

White Clover

Wild Carrot

Wild Carrot (Daucus Carrot) sometimes called of our country roads in Summer. Poisonous plant can pop up where they are least expected. All part of the plants are poisonous especially the seed - especially the seeds which are covered in a thorny case. It smells foul which should deter people and animal from eating in.

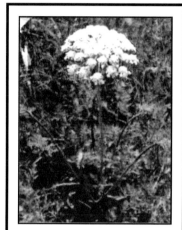

Wild Carrot

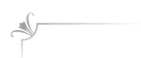

Cleavers

The most widespread of the Calium Species is Cleavers or goose-grass (Calium aparine) a Cosmopolitan weed that grows throughout the Northwest. It is a weak-stemmed. Branched annual with hooks on the angles of the square stem. It uses these hooks to help scramble over other vegetation. The leaves grow in whorls to 6 to 8 that radiate from the stem, like the spokes of a weel. They are about an inch long, elliptical, have a single conspicuous vein and are sharp-pointed, but not spiny, the tiny white flowers appear in branched inflorescences. The four petal of each flower fuse at the base into a short, narrow tube. The fruit are constricted parallel to the stalk, forming what appears to be matched pair of miniature nut. Hooked bristles densely cover these nutlets and aid in the dissemination of the two enclosed seed. Cleavers grow in wide range of habitas, from open forest to sunny weste??? areas. Usually it is associated with other weed, species which it uses for support. Forming an ungainly tangle of rank vegetation.

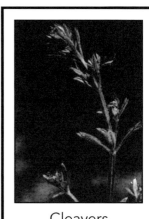

Cleavers

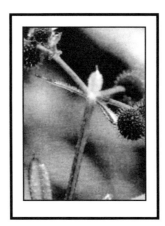

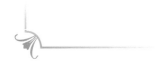

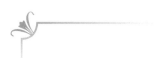

– D –

Dandelion

Members of this large subfamily share two outstanding characteristics that distinguish them from ALL other plants in the sunflowers, and bruised or torn beed milky juice. Most species have yellow ray but there are exception most produce seed with a parachute-like pappus which aids in seed dispersal. The group includes numerous weedy species, none more common than the ubiquitous dandelion.

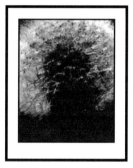 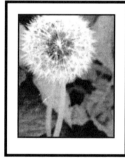 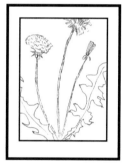

Dandelion

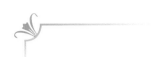

Dock

There are a few common weedy the seed can survive in the soil for up to century. In a recent study in the UK, dock seeds were found in small samples of soil a third of the gardens tested.

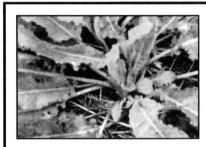

Dock

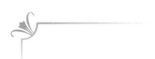

Dack Leaf
Smart Weed

This an erect, branched annual the papery sheaths above flower are pale green. This Eurasian weed most common branched annual with rather long (2 to 5 inches), lance shaped leaves. The papery sheaths above the leaves have slender, soft bristles around the tip. Flower are pale green to pinkish and grow in cluster at stem tip. This European weed most commonly infests irrigated field and gardens.

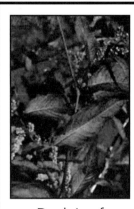

Dack Leaf

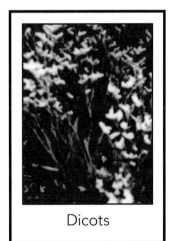

Dicots

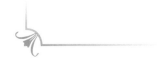

Douglas Mugwort

Tree of the most widespread and weedy species of the Northwest are absinth wormwood (Artemisia absinthium) a European an weed with finely divided leave common Mugwort (A vulgaris), also a European weed with divided, wooly leaves and Douglas Mugwort (A douglasiana) properly a hybrid with narrowly elliptical leaves, which are wooly beneath and in some plants divided.

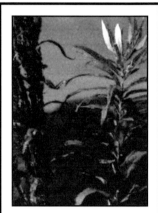

Douglas Mugwort

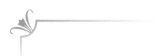

Diffuse knpweed

It is a biennial herb that grows from a slender taproot. The diffusely branched stem gives the plant a rounded profile after the seeds mature, the stem become dry and brittle and break off at ground level, making the plant a tumbleweed. The leaves are pinnatly divided, frequently into small segment; the upper ones are much reduced in size and less divided than the lower leaves. Each plant produce numerous narrow head, about ¾ of an inch wide. The overlapping involucral bracts are especially onate; they are spine-tipped and both sides are fringed with bristles, the flower are cream-colored to lavender. Rays are absent and the outer disc flower are not enlarged.

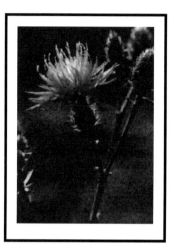

This species was introduced from Asia Minor early 1900s perhaps in alfalfa seed. It is now especially abundant in Central Washington and adjacent British Columbia, ranging South into Northern Oregon and West through Idaho into Western Montana. It is most abundant in disturbed areas but regularly invades grassland, threatening natural communities.

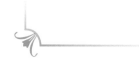

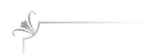

Fennal (Foeniculum Vulgare)

Is a flowering plant species in the Carrat family. It is hardy perennial herb with yellow flower and feathery leave. It is indigenous to the shores of the Mediterranean but has became widely naturalized in many parts of world, especially dry soils near the Sea-Caas and on riverbanks. It is highly aromatic and flavorful herb used in cookery and, along with the similar tasting anise, is one of the primary ingredients of absinthe Florence fennel or finocchio. Fennel is used as food plant by the larvae of some Lepidoptera Sepecies including in native??? mouse moth and the old world swallowtail. Where it has been introduced in North America it my by used by anise swallowfull.

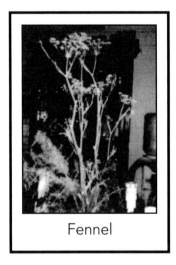
Fennel

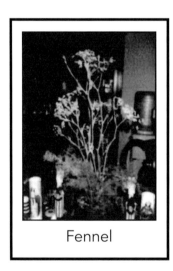
Fennel

Etymology and names

The word fennel developed from Middle English fennal or feny??? come from old English penol or finol, which in turn come from Latin feniculum or faeniculum the diminutive of fenum??? aenum meaning hay the Latin word for the plant was ferula which is now used as genus name of related plant fennel was prized the ancient Greek and who used.

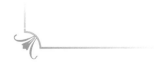

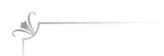

Fenugreek. ???

Fenugreek. Methi; Trigonella foenum graecum) is an annual plant in the Fabaceae with leaves consisting of three small obovate to oblong leaflets. It is cultived worldwide as semiarid crop. Its seeds and leaves are common ingredients in dishes from the Indian subcontinent where it is called Methi. Also used in traditional medicine, fenugreek (Methi), can increase the risk for serious medical side effects, though its culinary use (in smaller quantities) is usually believed to be safe. Fenugreek is not approved or recommended for clinical use by any government health agency.

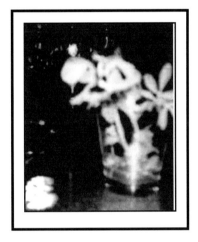

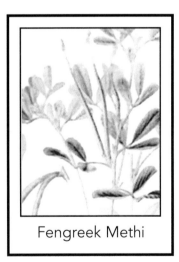

Fengreek Methi

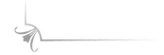
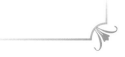

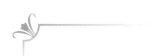

Foxtail

Yellow foxtail and bristly foxtail are fast growing grasses that thrive in cultivated soil waste places and in arable crop. Bristly foxtail has barbed seed and gets stuck in animal fur. There are several other similar species.

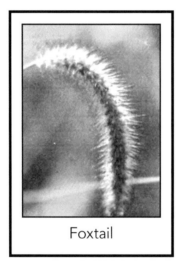

Foxtail

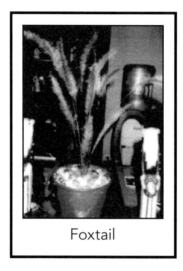

Foxtail

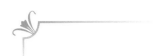

Field Mastard

Field Mastard typical member of the genus, has large, pinnatly compound basal leaves, with the terminal leaf segment larger than the others. The stem leaves lack stalk (petioles) and are rather ear-like in appearance. With two ear lobes extending from the stem opposite the leaf blade. The showy bright yellow flower have petals approximately ½ inch long, and continue to blossom at stem tip after the lower flower have matured into pod-like fruits. The fruit are approximately 2 inch long narrow, and have a beak-like tip. They seplit open at maturity to release the seed. A European weed field mastard is now widely distributed in North America, growing primarily in wease places and in cultivated fields like the cultivated species.

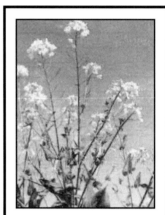

Field Mastard

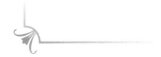

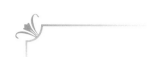

– G –

Bunch grass

Bunch grass community in Palouse Country of Washington State. Shows domination by weed especially fancy mustard and cheat grass, with the complete exclusion of native bunch grasses. These weed established themselves in 1941 when the field was abandoned. They still persist after nearly 50 years!

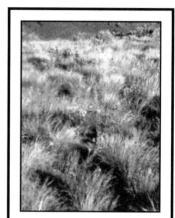

Bunch Grass

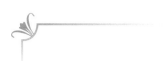

Grab Grass

This annual weed spreads horizontally, carb like, over the ground in a near circular pattern. Each spreading stem terminates in three to five finger-like branches. The spikeles are more or less pressed against these branches. The generic name is derived from Latin digitus, relating to this digitate or finger-like originally native of Europe. This grass has now become a Cosmopolitan weed. A closely related species of Grab Grass, Digitaria. Introduced wide-ranging weed in North America.

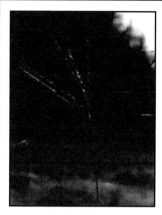

Grab Grass

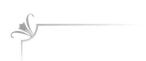

Groundsel.

Although it is member of the daisy family. The is on of the least attractives each flower actually a collection of tiny, individual flowers. Lack the usual ring of large outer flowers or petals.

Groundsel hybridized with the alienen Oxford ragwort to give rise to Welsh groundsel. Cambrensis. A new species and on of the UK very few endemic plants.

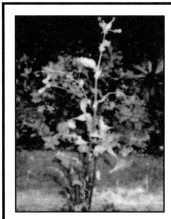

Groundsel

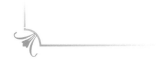

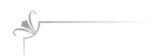

Giant Hogweed

Another weed that like Japanese knotweed started out as garden plant. However giant hogweed is rarely a problem in garden although its a very troublesome weed in the wider countryside is possibly the tallest herbaceous plant in Europe.

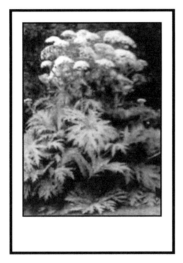

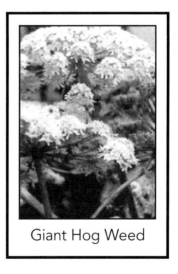

Giant Hog Weed

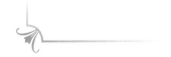

Grasses

Grasses a group that includes the bamboos inceasinly popular garden plant. Many of them are well behaved but some are not.

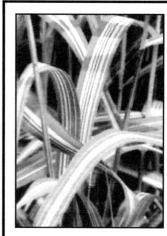

Grasses

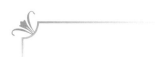

Green AmaranthAramanth

Now hailed as super green. Aramanth is a nutritious weed also known as pig weed. Common weed on lighter soils such as in East Anglia. And often appear where the soil is enriched, for example by big manure, which my be why it is also called pigweed. It is a very good food source for birds, who love a seed. But we can eat it too. Aramanth is another edible green, quite mild in flavour and usually found in the warmer month. In Greece it is cooked and dressed with olive oil and lemon juice, and it's common food in South India. The seed are small, but they are said to be high in protein, and there are various recipes for making a porridge from them Aramanth. It's suggested that it might replace kale as trendy vegetable for chefs steam or blanch it don't cook it for long and serve it like spinach.

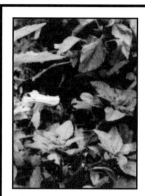

Green Aramanth

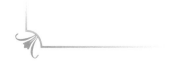

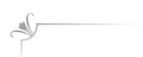

Hoary Gress White Top

White hairy (hoary) Gress perennial spreads through rhizomes forming denes clones. The stems are about a foot tall, with several branches bearing dense clusters of small white flowers responsible for the frequently used common name of white top. The branches are of nearly equal height, giving the plant a flat-topped appearance, the fruits look like small inflated hearts, the toothed leaves clasp the stem and have ear like lobes. This European species is becoming a noxious weed in much of North America.

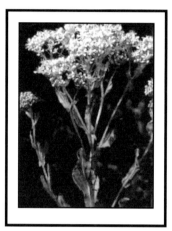

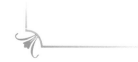

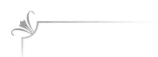

Hors Weed

Hors weed definitely is not attractive. It is hairy annual herb from, growing a few inches to a few feet tall. The single stem branches diffusely above, producing numerous very small head. The white rays are minute and inconspicuous, numerous, narrow leaves extend up to the head. Although horseweed is a native, it is an opportunistic weed thriving in disturbed areas over much of North America.

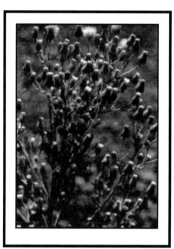

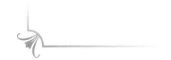

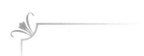

Giant Hours Tail

Horsetails are recognized by their succulent, hollow, jointed stems with terminal spore-producing cones, have separate reproductive stems the form are flesh-colored, lack branches, and appear in early in the spring before associated vegetation has grown tall. Tall enough to interfere with wine flow. The green vegetative stems. Slender branches are North America Houres common Hors tail the sterile stem 6-18 inches tall and exceeding 6 feet in high in the west.

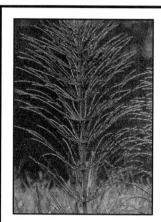

Giant Houres Tail

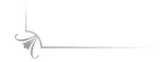

Poison Ivy (Sumag family) Rhusradicans Poison Ivy my not deserve to be called a weed since it is not particularly invasive and is native to North America. However, it frequently forms rather dense thickets and is a common inhabitant of dry open forests, it grows especial. Well along some of our major river drainages. Undoubtedly it would escape the derogatory connotation of weed if its toxic oil did not cause a burning or itching rash on people allergic to them. Two North-Western species of Rhus cause dermatitis; poison ivy and poison oak they are distinguished primarily by their leaves. The three leaflets of poison ivy are generally not lobed and rather sharply pointed. The very small flowers are dull white and inconspicuous in elongate clusters.

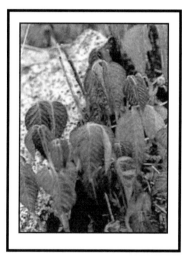

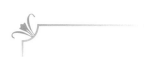

Indian Balsam

Indian Balsam. Indian or Himalayan balsam (Impatiens glanduliferra). A plant introduced to Britain in 1839 for it's. It grows rampant along some of our river systems, changing the ecology of river bank. Many other plant were brought to Britain by plant, haunter looking for new fashion in gardening. Originally much admired some have become weed.

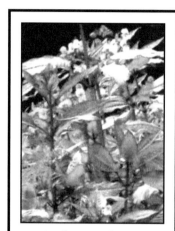

Indian Balsam

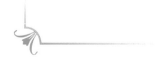

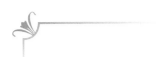

St. Johns-Wort

St. Johns Wort family the several erect stems of this perennial herb. The leaves are elliptical and opposite, about an inch long, and have black glandular dots along the margin. The very attractive flowers have five bright yellow petals, five sepals, and numerous purple-tipped stamens that project from the other floral parts. Deep purple dote along the jagged edges enhance the showiness of the ½ inch petals. The fruit is a many-seeded, woody capsule. The species name refers to the purplish dots that appear to perforte the leaves and flowers.

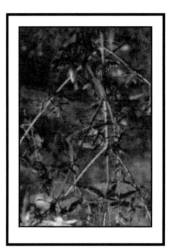

San Johans-Wort is one of most aggressive and noxious weed in the North West. It grow most conspicuously along roadsides, but regularly invades prairies meadows and pastures, where it successfully competes with more desirable plant. Crazing promotes the establishment of this unpalatable and, reputedly, mildly poisonous weed. It reproduces primarily by seeds but spreads also by short rhizomes. St. John-Wort is now being controlled to some extent by a leaf feeding beetle, in successful application of biological weed control. Like so many nasty weed, this is European import that now range over much of North America

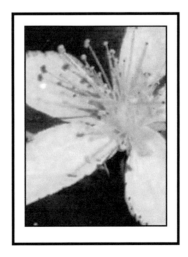

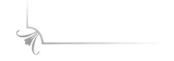

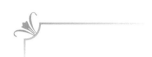

– K –

Diffus Knap Weed

It is a biennial herb that grows from a slender taproot. The diffusely branched stem give the plant arounded profile. After the seeds mature, the stem become dry and brittle and bresk off at ground level, making the plant tumbleweed. The leaves are pannately divided, frequently into small segments; the upper ones are much reduced in size and less divided than lower leaves. Each plant produces numerous narrow head, about 314 of an inch wide. The flower are cream-colored to lavender. Outer disc flower are not enlarged. This species was introduced from Asia Minor early in the 1900s. Perhaps in Alfalfa seed.

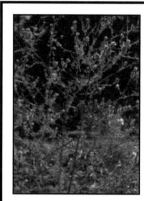

Diffus Knap Weed

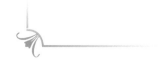

Knotgrass

Despite it's a common name, knotgrass is - clearly not a grass. In fact, it is a small mostly prostrate weed that is an annual relative of Japanese knotweed. Has tiny flower knotgrass but larger. More bindweed like leaves.

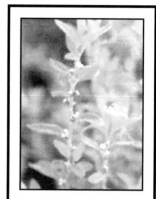

Knotgrass

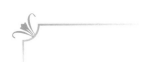

Common Knotweed

Common knotweed is prostrate plan that forms widely spreading mats flower are very small, green to reddish in color, and grow in small clusters in leaf axils leaves are also small and elliptical in outline. This ubiquitous weed infests a variety of habitas, from weaste areas to lawns, often in compacted trampled. It was introduced from Europe.

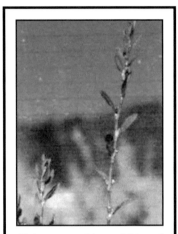

Common Knot Weed

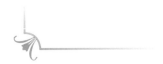

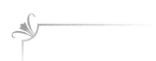

Lamb's Quarters Pig Weed

This is an extensively branched. Ungainly annual, 1 to 3 feet tall. The leaves are triangular or more or less diamond-shaped with lobed margins. The Latin name relates to the shape of the leaves: chen=goose, podium=foot album reflect the whitish coloration imparted by mealy material scattered over the plant. The tiny, individually indistinct, greenish flower densely cluster along branch tip. Lamb's quarter is a ubiquitous weed, occurring regularly in cultivated field, wasteland, and gardens. It is edible: the leaves can be used as a salad green, and the plants can be prepared as a potherb some domestic animals especially pigs, favor it is somewhat salty flavor, thus the name pigweed. It is a native of Eurasia.

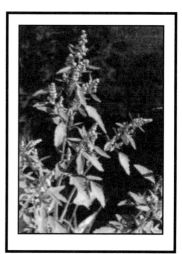

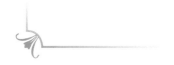

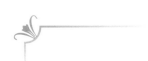

Russian Knapweed

This species is another candidate for most noxious knapweed. It is an aggressive perennial that spread from deep rhizom to form dense population. The extensively branched stems produce numerous head. The upper lower leaves are small and narrow; the large lower leaves are about 5 inches long. 2 inches across, and toothhead or lobed, the head are about half an inch wide and high; the involucral bracts have paper like tip and margins that are neither fringed nor spiny. The flowers are pink to purple and marginal once are not enlarged. This plant was introduced from Turkestan about the turn of the century. It tolerate drought, and now grow throughout much of the Northeran Great Besin and into Canada.

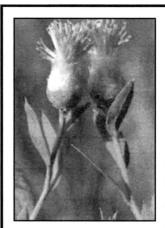

Russian Knapweed

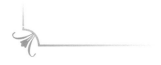

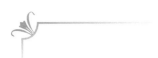

Leafy Spurge

This three feet tall perennial spreads by rootstalks as well as by seeds. The lower leaves are narrowly strap-shaped and about two inches long. The upper leaves near the flowers, are opposite and broadly heart shaped. The yellow floral bracts resemble a set of miniature but stout horns a noxious weed in much of the northern United State and adjacent Canada. This European import invades rangeland as well as wasteland. It is massive number of seed and very deep rhizomes makes it extremely difficult to eradicate.

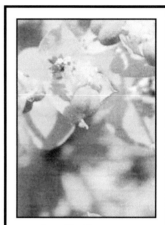

Leafy Spurgs

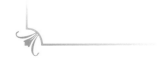

Prickly Lettuce

Biennial herb. The generic name Lactuca Latin for milk. Refer to this plant as milkweed. The plants 2 to 4 feet tall, with leafy stem and a as starchy taproot. The leaves are pinnately divided or sometime only toothed. They clasp the stem and have ear-like lobes. Prickles cover the leaf teeth. Lower surface of midven, and the lower half stem, thus the common name. Numerous narrow head grow on thin branches near the stem tip. The involural bract are very uneven in length and surround 6 to 8 lemon-yellow flower. The rays are about ⅓ inch long and finely toothed at the tip. The seeds are teardrop shaped but have a long thread-like crown which bears the parachute-like papus. This European native now grow over much of North America. It is common weed of waste places. Prickly Lettuce varies toward cultivated lettuce.

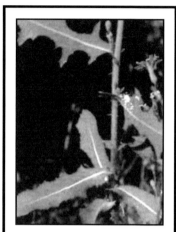

Prickly Lettuce

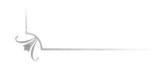

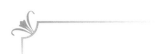

– M –

Tansy Mustard

Three weedy species of Desurania grows in the Northwest they are difficult to distinguish and occupy similar habitats. All are branched annuals with pinnately divided leaves, the leaf lobes further divided or toothed stems and leaves are covered with minut staar like hairs and are sometimes glandular hairy as will. The very small yellow flowers are than ¼ inch wide and rather inconspicuous the fruits are narrow pods, ¼ to ¾ inch long that project upward paralleled to the stem. D. Sophia was introduced from Europe to become the worst weed of the three species. The other are native to North America. Tansy mustards abound in wasteland and abused prairies to the detriment of native grasses.

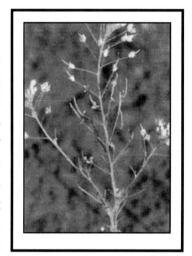

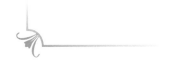

Black Mustard

This species resembles field mustard in general appearance, but is distinguishable on the basis of the stem leaves and fruits. The stem leaves are generally stalked, and not ear-like at the base; the fruits grow upward parallel to the stem instead of projecting perpendicular to it. Black mustard also tends to be more robust and more extensively branched than field also tends to be more robust and more extensively branched than field mustard. It is another European native that has become a ubiquitous weed in North American growing along roadsides, in waste places, and in field, both cultivated and abandoned.

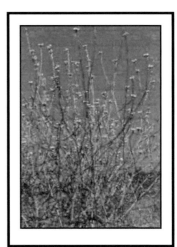

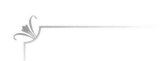

Common Mullein

One of the most conspicuous weed along the highway of the Northwest, Mulleins dry branched from superficially resembles a Saguaro Cactus. The species is a coarse biennial. In the first year it grows a low rosette of densely wooly leaves and a thick taproot. The rosette leaves may be more than a foot long and half as wide. They are nether, lobed nor toothed. The second year a single erect 2 to 4 foot stem grows from the tap root. The lower leaves are large and have long stalk. The upper leaves are smaller and stalkless. The flowers grow in dense, narrow clusters along the upper part of the main stem and shorter branches. The yellow petals are fused into

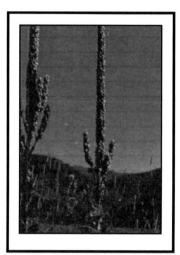

a short tube with five spreading lobes after shedding their seed. The plants die. But standing as silent as silent sentinels across the dry and desolate landscape mullein is noticeable weed. Such as roadsides.

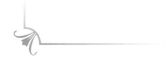

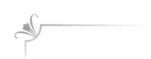

Common Mullein

One of most conspicuous weed along the highway of Northwest, Mullein's dry, branched from superficially resembles a Saguro Cactus. The species is coarse biennial. In the first year in grow a low rosette of densely wooly leaves and thick taproot, the rosette leaves may more than foot long and half as wide. They neither lobed. The second year a single erect, 2 to 4 foot stem grow from the top root. The lower leaves are large and have long stalk, the upper leaves are smaller and stalkless, the flowers grow in dense, narrow clusters along the upper part of main stem and shorter branches. The yellow petals. Although mullein is noticeable weed. Disturbed area, such as road sides, native of Eurasia.

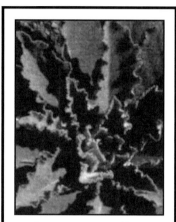

Common Mullein

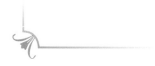

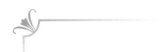

– M –

Mous ear chikweed

This sprawling, perennial herb root at the nodes, but has erect flowering stem. The egg-shaped leaves are opposite, crowded on the prostrate branches but rather widely spaced on the erect stems. Those on the ereat setem are larger, up to two inches and lack stalks. Hiars some of which are glandular and stick, cover both the leaves and stems. The small flower cluster at the tips of the erect stem this Eurasian weed common please, having become established over much of North America. It is especially invasive in lawn, pastures, cultivated field, and gardens.

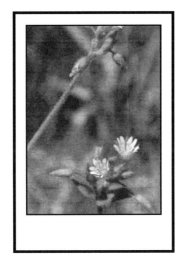

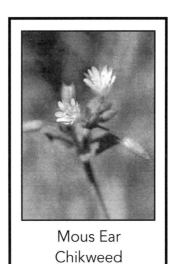

Mous Ear
Chikweed

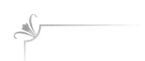

Monocts. Monocotyledon

Commonly referred to as monocots, (Lilianae sensu chase & Reveal) are flowering plants (angiosperms) the seed of which typically contain only one embryonic leaf, or cotyledon. They constitute on of the major groups into which the flowering plants have traditionally been dived, the rest of the flowering plant having two cotyledons and classified as dicotyledondons, or dicots, however, molecular phylogenetic research has shown that while monocots from a monophyletic group or clade. The

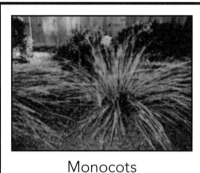

Monocots

dicotyledons do not. the monocotyledon include about 60,000 species the largest fome in this group.

Mallow

Mallow (Malya prviflora, M. Neglecta and other Malva species)

Mallow is often called marshmallow. True marshmallow Calthaea officinalis is a related plant used in medicine and traditionally to make marshmallow sweets, although modern recipes use gelatin.

Mallow is eaten by sheep and cattle, usually with no problem. However, cases of poisoning have occurred where animals particularly lambs have eaten mallow and nothing else which might the case if they were confind to small area. Can develop the condition called Staggers

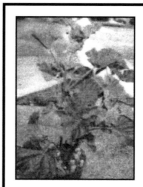

Mallow

– N –

Hairy Night Shad

Weak-stemmed and extensively branched. This hairy annule spread over the ground. The leaves are alternate and very from egg - to spear shaped, with bluntly toothed margins. The flower, similar in shape to those of the bittersweet nightshade, are dull white and not particularly showy the berry is pale green at maturity. Hairy night shade is a native of South America that has spread over much of North America. Including the North West. It is primarily a weed of cultivated fields and gardens.

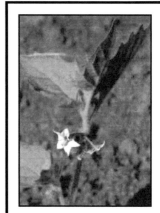

Hary Night Shad

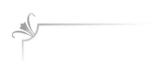

Bittersweet Nightshad

This nightshade has a persistent woody base and grows from rhizomes the vine-like stem scramble over other vegetation. The leaves very from entire and egg-shaped to trifolite and typically have two ear-like lobes at the base of the 1 to 3 inch blads. The flower grow on branches from short stalk that extands outward from the stem. The five blue-violet petal resemble a star with the point arching backward. The cone formed by the stamens is conspicuously yellow the ovary matures into bright red berr. The leaves and especially, the green fruit or moderately poisonous. The native of Eurasia is widespread in North America, where it grow in wast areas and along water ways and lake shores.

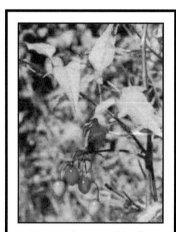

Bitter Sweet Night

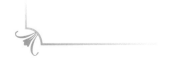

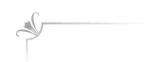

Nettle Curtica, Dioica, Urtica Urens)
Young nettle.

Up to about a hundred ago, nettle were grown in glass frames in Scotland to provide a green vegetable in early spring they knew about Vitamin C. people felt instinctively that they needed greens; several common weed had great value in winters when fresh food was scarce. It's almost commonplace now to hear people enthusing about nettle. When they are wilted or cooked they lose their sting, and they are extremely nutritious when young, nettle are very platable more than this, Nettle have many other uses and I love to hear from anyone who has tried them. The tough fibrous stem of taller kind were spun

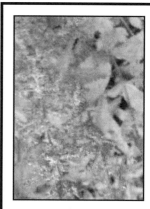

Nettle Seed

and woven to make a cloth-like linen for sheets and tablecloths. Nettle cloth was common in eighteen century houses. Like flax, the stem, had to be steeped in water to soften them the oily seed are said to have been used to fuel lamp; also in Shampoothe help to make the hair glossy. Some spinner and weaver use a soft green nettle dye for wool on plant dyes for more. Herb beers were popular in the nineteen century, and wear sometime made in an effort to wean the worker from alcoholic beer, which was astand household for centuries.

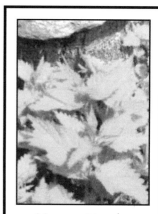

Young Nettle

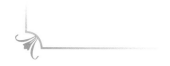

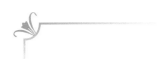

– O –

Orchard Grass

Orchard Grass is tall coarse perennial in introduced from Europe as a forage species. Each plant produces several 3 to 4 foot stems. Flat leaves approximately ¼ in wide. The way the spikelets are porne or stiff branches in denst one sided clusters.

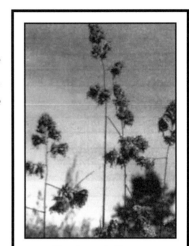

Orchard Grass

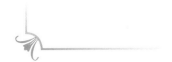

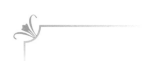

Oxalis or Shamrock

These weeds are also known as sorrels, but don't confuse them with true sorrels the herbs Rumex acetosa and R. Scutatus there are many weedy Oxalis, with yellow or pink flowers and they include some of the most intractable of all weed.

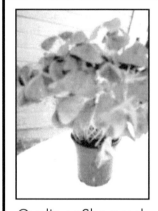
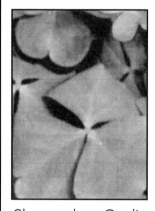

Oxalis or Shamrock   Shamrack or Oxalis

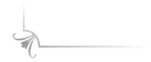

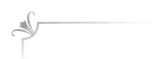

Oxeye daisy

This perennial herb spreads by rhizomes. The stem are rather stem are rather thin, 1 to 2 feet tall, and typically branch above to produce two or more attractive flower heads. The leaves are generally pinnately or divided the lower onces have rather long stalks the upper onces are stalkless and clasp the stems. The heads are about two inches across and have narrow bracts with brown, papery margins. The rays (15 to 30 per head) are pure white and the central disc flower are yellow. This plant was probably introduced from Europe as an ornamental. This species is now widespread in the North West and continues to increase its range.

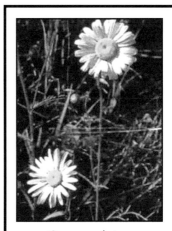

Oxeye daisy

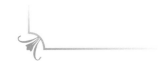

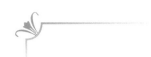

– P –

Poison Helock

This coarse, extensively branched, perennial grow to well over six feet. Purplish-red splotches mark the hollow stems. The larger leaves many be as much as foot long. All leaves are parsley-like and have enlarged petioles that sheat the stem. Each plant has numerous unbels of very small white flowers. The mature fruit are elliptical. Strongly ridged, and hirless. This species is the hemlock of classical antiquity. It is deadly poisons known to be responsible for recent death. Poison heloch often grows profusely in moist wast areas. Purplish splotches on the stem. Grows of wast cascades. It was in 400 BC was introduced from Eurasia.

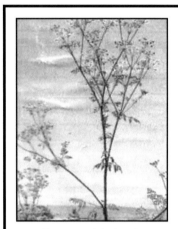

Poison Helock

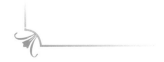

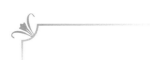

Pineapple Weed

Pineapple weed is branched, annual herb grows to about foot tall. The alternate leaves are twice or thrice pinnute, delicate and fern-like the leaves and stems are rather shiny and hairless. Numerous cone-shaped head are produced one the many branches. There are not ray flower and the tiny disc flower are yellow-green. The involuerl bracts are small and ovate, with papery margins. They are about half as long as head. This rather attractive plant has pleasant pineapple odor. Its an excellent substitute for chamomile in herb tea, but it not an aggressive weed native of North America.

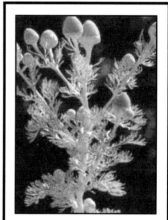

Pineapple Weed

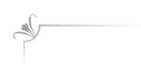

Redroot pigweed

Of the several species of Amaranthus that grow weeds in North Weast the most widespread is root this is an erect annual 1 to 3 feet tall, with long-stemmed, egg-shaped leaves the thick taproot is red as the common name suggest the minut flowers are individually surrounded by three bract and are densely clustered in several cone-shaped spikes. Thousands flowers my grow on each plant, each producing a single seed. Red is a pernicious weed of cultivated fields. Waste areas and gardens deal with especially when the bracts are dry. The generic name Amarnthus refer to the rigid persistence of these bract. Redroot is native of tropical America

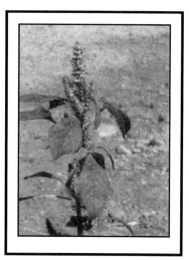

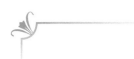

Poison Ivy Poison Oak

Poison Ivy may not deserve to be called a weed since it is not particularly invasive and is native to North America. However, it frequently forms rather dense thicktet and is common inhabitant or dry. Open forests. It grows especially well along some of our major river drainages. Undoubtedly it would escape the derogatory connotation of weed. If its toxic oils did not cause a burning or itching rash on people allergic to tham.

Poison Oak (R. diveriloba), they are distinguished primarily by their leaves. The three leaflets of poison ivy are generally shallowly-lobed and rounded at the tip. However the leaf shape overlap the very small flower are dull white and inconspicuous in elongate. The fruit are whitish berries. Have colorful red leaves in Autumn

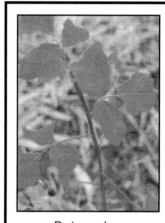

Poison Ivy

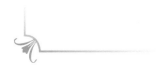

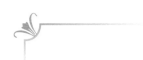

Corn Poppy

Poppy is often a weed of annual crops, winter, cereals, gardens, meadows, and disturbed sites. Crop losses of 43% has been reported. It is easily controlled by herbicides, but seed bank viability are concern. Similar species: Long-headed pony (p. dubiul) poppy. It is distinguished by red to orange petals up to 3 cm flower stalk with appressed long.

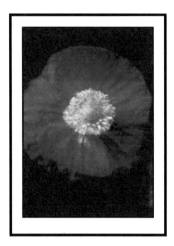
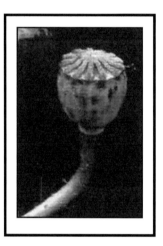

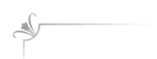

Pickle Weed
Pickle Grass

Saliccornia is genus of Succulent (salt-tolerant) flowering plant in family Amaranthaceae that grow in salt marshes, on beaches, and among mangroves Solicornia species are native to North America, Europe, South Asia common names for the genus include glasswort peickleweed peiclegrass and marsh samphire these common names are also used for some species not in Salicornia. To French speakers in Atlantic Canada, they are known, colloquially as titines de souris (mous tits) the main European species is often eaten, called pickle weeds marsh samphire in Britain, and the main North America

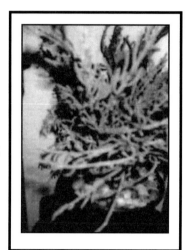

species is occasionally sold in grocery store or appears on restaurant meanus usually ass sea beans or samphire greens or sea asparagus.

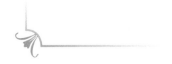

– Q –

Quack Grass

Quach grasses sometime called couch grass spreads by rhizomes forming a thick tough sod. The stems stand erect up to three feet tall and the leaves are long flat and about ⅓ in wide seipkelets with their flower grains and associated bracts.

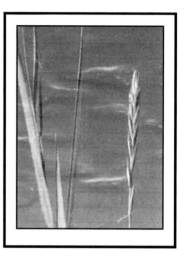

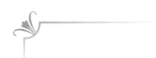

Queen Anne's Lace
Daucus Earota

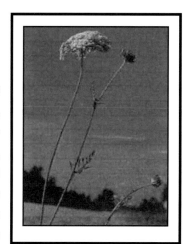

Queen Ann's Lace resembles the carrot, as well it should since it is wild carrot. It is an erect biennial, up to four feet tall, with lace-like, muticopound leaves. The plants are usually. Coasely hairy the carrot-like roots taste like their cultivated cousins but become woody, bitter and tough as the plant ages. The minut white flowers grow in a flat-topped inflorescence, technically a compound Umbel because it contains small Umbels within a large Umbel. The central flower is usually pinkish purple. Leaves immediately below the inflorescence are small but pinntely divided. Short bristles envelope the mature fruit fruits. When it blooming late summer, Queen Ann's Lace is one of the most common and conspicuous weed along roadsides in the Pacific Northwest. It thrives primarily in wast areas but invades meadows and and pastures. It is native of Eurasia.

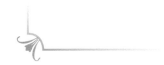

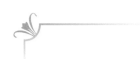

– R –

Ragwort

A tall biennial producing a large clabbage like rosette of ragged or divided leaves in its first year and prodigious quantities of very effectively wind dispersed seeds in its second.

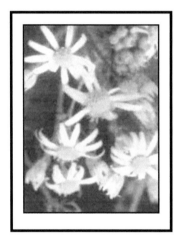 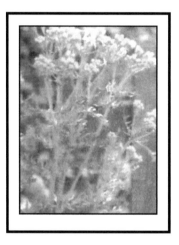

– S –

Shamrock

These weeds are also known as Sorrels, but don't confuse them with true Sorrels the herbs Rumex acetosa and R. Scutatus there are many Weedy Oxalis, with yellow or pink flowers and they include some of the most intractable of all weed.

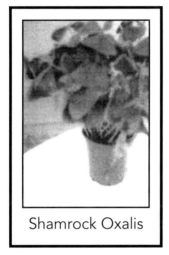

Shamrock Oxalis

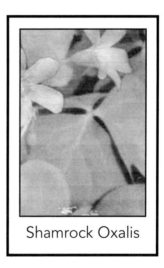

Shamrock Oxalis

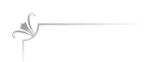

Scarlet Pimpernel

Tiny weeds such a scarlet (Anagallis arvenisis) help to cover dry ground. This is a native annual, dying down each year after producing seed. There is also a blue form, equal attractive, which is found in Spain and other places with plenty of sunshine. The flower only open in good weather - it's coutrymans barometer and only from about nine in the morning to three in afternoon. I had to watch carefully to get a photograph, because when the flower are closed they are hidden in the leaves.

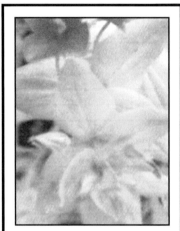

Scarlet Pimpernel

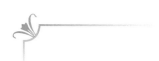

Spurges

Spurges all have tiny greenish flowers surrounded by conspicus bract. These two weed species are annuals. But many perennial euphorbias are grown as garden plant.

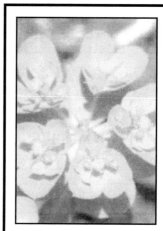

Spurges

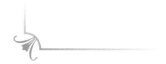

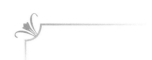

– T –

Cotton Thistle Scotch Thistle

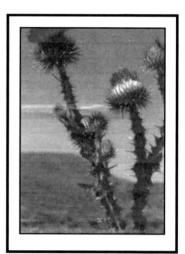

Cotton thistle is the granddaddy of the thistles; it may grow much as nine feet tall. It is an extensively branched biennial herb, conspicuously clotted in cottony hairs and covered by vicious, yellowish spines. The stems and branches have prominent spiny pleats that resemble long, thin fine. These wings continue down from the bases of alternate leaves, which are about a foot long and half as wide. The leaves are coarsely and irregularly toothed; spines tip the teeth. Spine-tipped, cottony involueral bracts surrounded the 1 to 2 inch wineheads flowers are reddish-purple. Onopordon is the ancient Greek word for thistle. This weed, a native of Europe, has been widely introduced at mid-latitudes across much of North America. In the North West, it is most troublesome along the Snake River drainage. It is sufficiently drought tolerant to invade grassland and sagebrush communities, especially were disturbed.

Sow Thistle (Sonchus Oleraceus)

Sow thistle (also milk thistle) sometimes appears are the edges of paddocks; it is a soft thistle with a small yellow flower and a milly sap in the hollow stem. It's not a true thistle, but like the thistle family it has a long tap root and high mineral content. We have both this from and the more prickly type (S. asper).

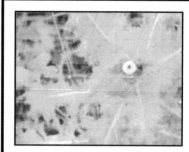
Sow Thistle

Thistle

Of this group of plant is of course, the spininess of the involucre bracts and, usually, of the leaves and stems. The large and showy heads lack ray flower, but the outer disc flowers are somewhat ray-like and often enlarged the group includes many of the most anxious weed in the Northwest. The combination of spinniess and aggressiveness places the thistle other thistle-like plants among our most hated weed. However, thistles have very attractive head that are subjects of painting the word over. The produce large amount of nectar and pollen. Food for variety of insects especially bumblees and butterflies. The late summer flowering time of many thistle plant ensures a nectar.

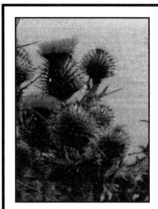
Thistel

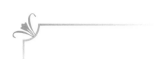

Teasel

Is rosette of leave that live. Coarse biennial herb the first year's growth is rosette of leaves that live through the winter. The following year a single erect stem emerges from the whorl of leaves, and grow to six feet tall. It is marked by longitudinal redges and minature spines. The leaves are opposite, lance-shaped, and up to a foot long. Generic name in Greek, dipsa, means thirsty. The leaves are prickly, especially along the midvein. The pale blue flower grow in denes thick spike at the stem tip. At the base of spike are several elongate bracts that are spiny in moist areas. Teasel can be a truly noxious weed. Desirable plants. It is common in waste areas and along road sides. The dry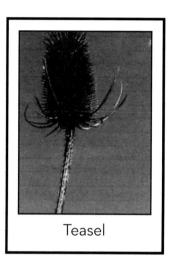

Teasel

spine flower stalk are frequently used decoration. Especially at Christmas. This European species. Is now widespread in North America.

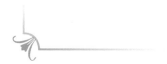

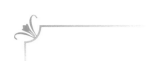

Thistle

Of this group of plant is of course, the spininess of the involucral bracts and, usually, of the leaves and stems. The large and showy heads lack ray flower, but the outer disc flowers are somewhat ray-like and often enlarged the group includes many of the most anxious weed in the Northwest. The combination of spinniess and aggressiveness places the thistle other thistle-like plants among our most hated weed. However, thistles have very attractive head that are subjects of painting the word over. The produce large amount of nectar and pollen. Food for variety of insects especially bumblees and butterflies. The late summer flowering time of many thistle plant ensures a nectar.

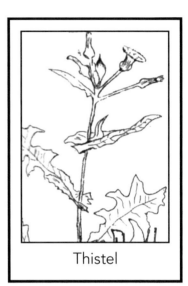

Thistel

Tansy Ragwort
Senecia Jacobaea

This renegade weed is a short-lived perennial herb that grows from a taproot to a height of about three feet. The stems are typically unbranched up to the spreading, flat-tapped inflorescence, which consist of several flower head. Each head, abulone inch across, displays 10 to 15 yellow rays and approximately as many disc flowers. The leaves are pinnately divide, rather carrot-like; the lower ones have long stalks, the above lack stalks Tansy Ragwort is a poisonous plant with a cumulative effect on. Tansy Ragwort on livestock in the pacific North West where the species is rapidly spreading, organized control efforts include the introduction of more or less host-specific herbrivous beetle. This native of European is now locally common in pastures and Western areas West of Casede rang.

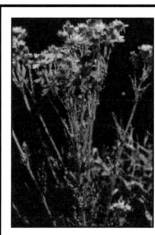

Tansy Ragwort

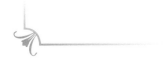

– V –

Vetchs

Are sometimes grown as animal fodder and can escape as weed, Lucene or alfafa. (Medicago Sativa), a cultivated type is often grown for feeding to cattle, just as it was by the ancient Greek and Romans. Lucerne hay is populas for horses. Deep roots, going down sometimes to 40 feet, protect Lucerne from dry weather, and it can be cut several times during the grazing season. Legumens are high in protein and weeds such as Vetch are good food for poultry and pigs.

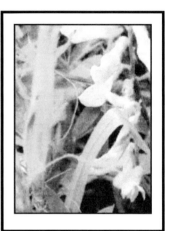

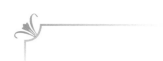

– W –

Wild Oat

Wild Oat is a tall 2-4 foot.
This wild cereal cosly resembles Oats but a long twisted, bristle like appendage are born on the back of one of the bracts, the own also assists in planting the seed grain when it absorbs moisture, it uncoils serving itself and the seed into soft soil of cultivated field.

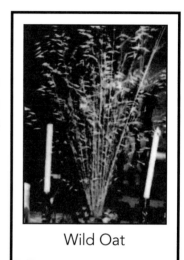

Wild Oat

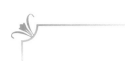

White Compion Fruits

This extensively branched, rather coarse perennial herb is covered
with short, soft hairs that become glandular stick on the flower
stalks. The leaves are opposite, the lower ones up to four inches
long and half an inch wide, the upper ones smaller. The ornate
petal divided into two major lobes with smaller appendage below.
The lower half of the petals is narrow and strap-like. The separates
fuse together into purple-striped the flower of the male plants are
somewhat show and the sepals have 10 purple stripes the sepals of
female flowers become much more infated and have 20 stripes. The
white divided flower like lamps in the night, attracted nectar moth

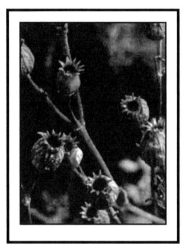

pollinators. Lychnos = lamps in Greek. A European plant ranges widely in North America. And
is therefore not considered a noxious weed.

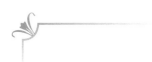

Watson's Willow herb

This is an extremely variable species both morphologically and ecologically. Although an herbaceous perennial that spreads from short rhizomes, it goes from seed to seed in single year like an annual. It may grow to over three feet tall under ideal condition of temperature and moisture, and branch extensively, under stressful condition, it usually grow to less than an foot, and remains unbranched. Flower and fruit production.

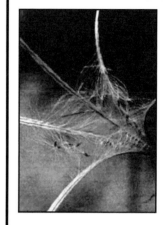

Vary similarly. The plants are usually hairy, often glandular. Leaves lack or nearly lack stalks. The lower ones are 1 to 3 inches long, opposite and lanceolate; the upper ones are smaller, alternate and egg-shaped. All leaves are more or less toothed. Flower vary in color from white to deep rose-purple and in size from ½ to ¾ inches across flower part comes in multiples of four. As is typical of willow-herbs, the ovary matures into a capsule 1 to 4 inches long that produce thousands of tiny seed each with a tuft of cottony hair, like those of the fireweed, the seeds disappear on the wind. Spread over the United States and has invaded Europe. Grows in rather moist waste areas.

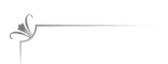

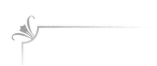

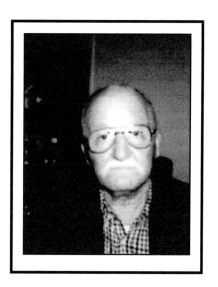

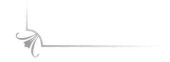

Printed in the United States
by Baker & Taylor Publisher Services